RHEUMATOID ARTHRITIS - The Simple Anti-Inflammatory Recipe Book for a Healthy Immune System.

28 Day Meal Plans

By Ross Lennox

CONTENTS

INTRODUCTION

As a sufferer of Rheumatoid Arthritis I realized early on that there was a direct link between the foods I was eating and the way I was feeling. The adoption of an anti-inflammatory diet and some simple changes in your shopping and eating habits could make a huge difference to your wellbeing, boost your energy levels, improve your confidence and impact on your pain and discomfort levels.

This book is simply designed to highlight some of the foods that can usefully be included in your weekly shopping that can really make a difference to the RA sufferer. We all know the importance of eating more fruit and vegetables, but some of these can offer higher levels of anti-inflammatory effects, and our shopping choices need to reflect this.

After this I have provided some easy to follow meal plans with delicious recipes all made using foods which will be kind to our bodies and help to reduce our RA symptoms. The adoption of an anti-inflammatory diet, whilst it will not cure the RA, can have a huge impact on how you personally feel. Making the right nutritional choices can have a major impact on how you feel both mentally and physically.

I wish you success in adopting an anti-inflammatory diet and hope it will being you the relief and a sense of positivity it has given to me.

Ross Lennox

CHAPTER ONE

Nutrition Recommendations for People with Rheumatoid Arthritis

While there's really no specific cure for those suffering from Rheumatoid Arthritis, meticulous meal planning can help you manage the symptoms. It is normal that those with RA are constantly looking for ways to help them manage the pain. According to studies, there's a connection between inflammation and certain foods that define this autoimmune condition.

The best nutrition for RA sufferers – or anyone else – is a well-balanced diet. Your daily meals should be centered on plant-based ones especially if you're trying to lose weight. Your diet should also comprise of whole grains, fruits, vegetables, lean sources of protein, and low-fat dairy products.

The Following are the Best Foods for People with Arthritis and they have an Anti-Inflammatory Effect:

Fish – this is packed with omega 3 fatty acids that help fight inflammation. According to experts, it is recommended that you eat fish at least twice a week. Some of the best fish to eat includes tuna, salmon, herring, and mackerel.

Garlic –those who regularly eat garlic, onion, and leeks show less signs of osteoarthritis. A compound called diallyl disulphine helps limits enzymes that damage the cartilage in human cells.

Beets – These are known to be chockfull of antioxidants that help repair cell damage mainly caused by inflammation. They have high levels of potassium and magnesium, which are known to fight inflammation.

Bok Choy – this is also known as Chinese cabbage and is considered to be rich in antioxidants, vitamins, and minerals. According to studies, there are at least 70 antioxidant phenolic substances found in this vegetable. So this is a great one to include in your weekly shopping list.

Broccoli – this vegetable has loads of health benefits for the body. It is rich in calcium, vitamins C, and K, which according to research, help in preventing osteoarthritis progression.

Celery – This has both anti-inflammatory and antioxidant properties that improve cholesterol levels and blood pressure. The seeds contain amazing health benefits and can aid in lowering inflammation and bacterial infections.

Cherries – when it comes to fruits, it is best to stock up on fruits like cherries, blueberries, raspberries, strawberries, and blackberries.

Citrus fruits – these are rich in vitamin C that prevent arthritis inflammation and in keep the joints healthy. Some examples are grapefruit, lime, and oranges.

Low fat dairy products – such as milk, cheese, and yogurt are filled with calcium, which is known to strengthen the bones and vitamin D, which helps boost one's immune system.

Soy – tofu or edamame – all these soy products are high in fiber and protein, and provide similar anti-inflammation benefits like omega 3 fatty acids.

Walnuts –These protects against type 2 diabetes, metabolic syndrome, and even heart disease. Walnuts are also rich in omega-3s and protein. This is one of those anti-inflammatory snacks that you can easily grab and munch on.

Chia seeds – These are an anti-inflammatory and antioxidant powerhouse that contain omega-3 and omega-6, vitamins A, B, E, and D, essential fatty acids such as linoleic acid and alpha-linolenic, strontium, and mucin, and important minerals including iodine, manganese, iron, magnesium, thiamine, and niacin. These seeds have the power to reverse inflammation, lower blood pressure, and regulate cholesterol levels.

Beans – these are chockfull of fiber and protein that help with muscle health and growth. Specifically look for pinto beans, red beans, and kidney beans as they are rich in magnesium, iron, zinc, and folic acid.

Flaxseeds – these are a great source of phytonutrients, antioxidants, and omega-3s. Polyphenols found in flaxseeds aid in probiotics' growth in the gut. To maximize its effectiveness, grind seeds in a coffee maker first.

Green tea – this is believed to have antioxidants that slow down the damage of cartilage and blocks molecule production, damaging the joints of those with RA.

Coconut oil – This reduces inflammation and helps in healing arthritis. Also, coconut oil helps fight free radicals and oxidative stress known to be the main culprits of osteoporosis.

Ginger – whether you use the supplement, fresh, or dried, ginger is considered to reduce inflammation and helps boosts one's immune system. This is also known to purify the lymphatic system and breaks down toxins in the major organs of the body. In fact, ginger helps in treating inflammation in both asthmatic and allergic conditions.

What about mayonnaise?
To avoid health disadvantages of store-bought mayonnaise, it is advised that you make your own using healthier oils such as olive and avocado oil. This way, you also get to control what you put in your mayonnaise and avoid artificial ingredients. A classic one often includes oil, egg yolks, vinegar, and seasonings. For gourmet versions, you may add in garlic, curry powder, or pesto.

What about Honey?

The use of honey for Rheumatoid Arthritis has showed amazing results. Honey has gained popularity in minimizing joint inflammation and for its antibacterial properties. Many people who are suffering from arthritis use this, there are lots on the market so why not try a few. Manuka honey is worth seeking out, and use honey as a natural sweetener.

Is baking soda allowed?
This is another effective treatment for rheumatoid arthritis whether you choose to dissolve it in water and drink it or add it as ingredient to your dishes. Baking soda helps in neutralizing the acidic condition of the body by raising the PH level. Those who are suffering from rheumatoid arthritis are acidic. The alkalinity property of the baking soda has the ability to dissolve uric acid crystals and helps relive joint pain.

Is milk allowed?

In truth, you really don't have to go dairy-free when you have arthritis since according to studies, there is no difference between RA patients who still drink milk and those that are on a dairy-free diet. In fact, when you drink milk, it fights osteoarthritis and prevents gout. If you are trying to lose weight, it is best that you opt for the low-fat or non-fat version.

Is Peanut butter allowed?

Use peanut butter as sauce for vegetables or chicken. If going grocery shopping, specifically look for organic peanut butter that list only 1 or 2 ingredients: peanuts and salt or peanuts only.

CHAPTER TWO

FOODS TO AVOID

Rheumatoid arthritis or RA is an inflammatory disease. What you eat affects how extreme or how often your flare ups will be. To avoid this, you may want to consider removing these foods that are deemed to cause flare ups:

Fried food – Deep-fried food such as potato chips, French fries, calamari, and even onion rings are high in food additives, trans fat, saturated fat, and sodium. All of which we could do with avoiding.

Trans Fats – this causes systemic inflammation and are mostly be found in processed snacks, frozen products, fast food, donuts, fried products, crackers, stick margarines, and cookies.

Saturated Fats – Some of the foods that trigger inflammation and worsen arthritis include pizza, red meat, pasta, full-fat dairy products, and sweet desserts.

Refined sugar – Did you know that the body's response to sugar intake is an increase in the production of stress hormones and insulin? These can greatly contribute to inflammation. So instead, try replacing them with complex carbohydrates such as whole grain bread, fruits, and vegetables. Eating fruit will not only help you manage your inflammation, but also help you control your sweet tooth.

Processed food – Fast food packaged meals are examples of overly processed food. These are loaded with food additives, sugar, unhealthy oils, and artificial flavors. Avoid calling for a fast food delivery or stopping at a drive thru, make it a habit to plan your meals for the week and have go-to snacks for when you're in a rush.

Sugar – processed ones found in sodas, chocolates, pastries, and even fruit juices can trigger the release of an inflammatory called cytokines. These are a large group of signaling molecules that are secreted by specific cells of the immune system and regulate inflammation, immunity, and hematopoiesis.

Salt – Too much salt can encourage inflammation. Processed foods are generally high in sodium. Those with lingering inflammatory conditions can benefit from a low sodium diet, preferably less than a teaspoon of salt or 1,500 mg a day.

Margarine – Trans fats found in margarine are considered a harmful ingredient and promote inflammation. Baked goods like biscuits, pies, and buns contain margarines and hydrogenated oils that are bad for people with rheumatoid arthritis.

Pork – arachidonic acid contained in red meat like pork are considered pro-inflammatory. Apart from this, processed pork products such as hotdogs, sausages, and bacon have added nitrates meant for color preservation that are found to also increase the risk of diabetes and heart diseases.

Beef – Fats from animals are mainly saturated fat. High-fat beef is linked to inflammation and has the possibility of altering the gut bacteria, which mainly causes immune response thereby stimulating inflammation.

White grain products – Some examples include pasta and breads that are made from refined grains. These quickly break down and convert into sugar, causing inflammation. Go for whole grains instead since they take longer to break down in the body.

Alcohol – excessive consumption can cause inflammation and weakens the proper function of the liver.

Grain Choices for Rheumatoid Arthritis Patients

To make the most out of nutrition while reducing inflammation, your diet should also consist of whole grains and those that are gluten-free. Some examples include:

Brown rice: This has not had the germ and bran stripped in the course of processing. This type of grain is best as a white rice replacement.

Quinoa: This high-protein grain is also another ideal substitute. According to research, quinoa may possibly defeat the release of cytokines, an immune substance that could be beneficial for treating and/or preventing inflammation.

Whole wheat: Swapping this for white flour will boost one's nutrient intake and could possibly lower inflammation.

Buckwheat-GF: This high-protein is technically a fruit but can be used as ingredient for pancakes, noodles, crepes, and muffins.

Millet-GF: This is a perfect alternative to rice, or added to recipes for muffins and bread.

Whole oats-GF: whole oats and steel-cut oats are high in protein, and are gluten free.

Barley: This is best for stews, risotto, and soups and contains 6 grams of fiber per cup.

Rye: If you're aiming to lose weight, this grain helps in suppressing one's hunger, so you can use it as ingredient for bread and other dishes.

Bulgur: This comes from whole-wheat and tastes like nuts. Use this in dishes just as you would couscous or rice.

Sorghum-GF: This grain is high in protein. The flour can be used as replacement for white flour in cookies, breads, and other dishes.

CHAPTER THREE
Suggested Joint-Friendly Grocery List for People with Rheumatoid Arthritis

Fish

- Sardines
- Trout
- Herring
- Salmon

Seeds

- Chia seeds
- Flaxseed
- Sesame seeds
- Hemp Seeds
- Walnuts
- Almonds

- Cashews nuts

- Macadamia nuts

Fruits

- Blackberries
- Strawberries
- Blueberries
- Black cherries
- Raspberries
- Oranges
- Peaches
- Papaya
- Grapefruit
- Kiwi

Vegetables

- Broccoli
- Bell peppers
- Brussels sprouts
- Cabbage
- Swiss chard
- Spinach
- carrots,
- asparagus
- cucumber
- beets
- celery
- kale
- parsley
- onions
- radish
- mushrooms

Beverages
- Green tea
- herbal tea
- Water infusions
- coconut water

Condiments
- sea salt
- peppercorns
- fresh herbs and spices

CHAPTER FOUR
Sample Weekly Meal Plan for 28 Days
Week 1

	Breakfast	Lunch	Snack	Dinner
Monday	Tofu Frittata	Loaded Vegetable Soup	Tuna and Avocado Ceviche on Jicama Slices	Mung Bean and Tomato Lettuce Wraps
Tuesday	Two Bean and Avocado Salad	Egg Noodle Tuna Casserole	All-Natural Power Berries Juice	Spicy Sardine-Stuffed Avocadoes
Wednesday	Coconut Butter on Vegan Rye Bread	Green Chili Peppers and Tomato Soup	Avocado Cream Cheese on Cucumber Slices	Tuna and Mango Salad
Thursday	Baked Apricot Oatmeal	Almond Baked Halibut Fillet	Oats and Dates Energy Bars	Seared Tuna
Friday	Red Berries Smoothie	Sardine and Garden Salad	Toasted Sesame Kale	Roasted Squash with Cranberries
Saturday	Granola Fruits and Nuts	Mackerel on Cucumber Sandwich	Twice-Baked Sweet Potatoes and Yam Matchsticks	Spiced Oriental Greens
Sunday	Dried Leaves Herbal Infusion & Berry Loaded Salad	Mung Beans and Tomato Lettuce Wraps	Baked Eggs in Avocado Halves with Wholegrain Sourdough Bread	Mediterranean-Style Tuna Salad

Week 2

	Breakfast	Lunch	Snack	Dinner
Monday	Egg Noodle Tuna Casserole	Quinoa-Stuffed Bell Peppers	Tropical Infusion	Barley Vegetable Soup
Tuesday	Arugula, Endive, and Radicchio Salad with Garlic Dressing	Sautéed Baby Zucchini	Tuna and Tomatoes Bread	Anchovy on Avocado and Salad Greens
Wednesday	Blueberries in Cream Cheese Flapjacks	Citrus Tuna Steaks	All Berries Sweetened Oats with Coconut Milk	Chilli Sweet Potatoes
Thursday	Two Bean and Avocado Salad	Country Cabbage Soup	Power Carrot Juice	Baked Zucchini with Mint
Friday	Vegetables Power Juice	Salmon and Dill Spread	Spiced Crisp Cauliflower	Spiced Eggplant
Saturday	Kale and Seeds Salad	Loaded Vegetable Soup	Coconut and Mangoes Flapjacks	Pickle and Potato Wraps with Miso Tahini Sauce
Sunday	Mixed Vegetable Soup	Butternut Pumpkin and Spinach Salad	Piña Colada Smoothie	Sesame Seared Tuna with Wasabi

Week 3

	Breakfast	Lunch	Snack	Dinner
Monday	Berry Cashew French Toast	Tuna Salad with Pickle Relish and Cheese	Tuna and Avocado Ceviche on Jicama Slices	Anchovy on Avocado and Salad Greens
Tuesday	Spinach and Strawberries Salad	Spiced Stir Fry Eggplant	Orange Water Infused with Cucumber and Grapes	Avocado and Salmon Stuffed Pita Bread
Wednesday	Mixed Greens and Blueberries Salad	Vegan Chili	Peach, Pineapple, and Mango Smoothie	Potato and Cauliflower Kadahi
Thursday	Apple Cinnamon Oatmeal	Baked Pineapple with Rice and Veggies	Lime Water Infused with Strawberries and Grapes	Tuna and Cucumber Salad
Friday	Greens with Sunflower Seed Salad	Pickle and Potato Wraps with Miso Tahini Sauce	Veggie Fritters	Green Chili Peppers and Tomato Soup
Saturday	Easy Boiled Plantains	Vegetable Relish	Citrus-Flavored Fruits and Vegetable Kebab	Sweet Potato Casserole
Sunday	Apples and Chamomile Herbal Infusion	Kidney and Garbanzo Beans Salad	Strawberry and Flaxseed Shake	Avocado and Salmon Stuffed Pita Bread

Week 4

	Breakfast	Lunch	Snack	Dinner
Monday	Power Berries Juice	Blueberry and Cashew Salad	Apple Cinnamon Oatmeal	Citrus Tuna Steaks
Tuesday	Tofu Frittata	Country Cabbage Soup	Tuna and Mango Salad	Kale and Seeds Salad
Wednesday	Blueberries in Cream Cheese Flapjacks	Tuna and Tomatoes Bread	Easy Boiled Plantains	Egg Noodle Tuna Casserole
Thursday	Power Carrot Juice	Green Chili Peppers and Tomato Soup	Shaved Fruits and Vegetables Infusion	Avocado and Salmon Stuffed Pita Brea
Friday	Peach, Pineapple, and Mango Smoothie	Almond Baked Halibut Fillet	Granola Fruits and Nuts	Quinoa-Stuffed Bell Peppers
Saturday	Baked Eggs in Avocado Halves with Wholegrain Sourdough Bread	Tuna and Cucumber Salad	Coconut Butter on Vegan Rye Bread	Roasted Squash with Cranberries
Sunday	Apples and Chamomile Herbal Infusion	Spiced Stir Fry Eggplant	Oats and Dates Energy Bars	Sardine and Garden Salad

Soup and Salad Recipes

Mixed Vegetable Soup

Ingredients:

- 1 tbsp. olive oil
- ¼ cup onion, chopped
- ¼ cup celery, chopped
- 1 can diced tomatoes, do not drain
- 2 cups frozen mixed vegetables, lightly thawed
- 2 cups vegetable broth
- 1 tbsp. sugar
- ¼ tsp ground marjoram
- 1/8 tsp pepper
- Seasoned salad croutons

Directions:

Pour olive oil in a saucepan. Saute onion and celery for 2 minutes or until tender.

Add in diced tomatoes, mixed vegetables, vegetable broth, sugar, ground marjoram, and pepper. Stir well.

Bring mixture to a boil.

Reduce the heat and allow to simmer for 20 minutes or until the veggies are tender.

To spread, garnish with salad croutons on top.

Green Chilli Peppers and Tomato Soup

Ingredients:

2 tbsp. olive oil

1 small onion, chopped

2 garlic cloves, minced

3 4 oz cans green chilli peppers, chopped

3 tbsp. ground cumin

4 14 oz can vegetable broth

28 oz can tomatoes, crushed

Pinch of salt

Pinch of pepper, to taste

1 avocado, diced

1 cup low fat cheddar cheese, shredded

Directions:

Pour olive oil in a large pan. Saute onion and garlic for 3 minutes or until fragrant and translucent. Add in green chili peppers and cumin. Cook for 3 minutes or until soft.

Pour vegetable broth and stir in tomatoes. Season with salt and pepper. Bring to a boil.

Once boiling, reduce the heat and allow to simmer for 30
minutes.

To serve, garnish with avocado and shredded cheese top.

Loaded Vegetable Soup

Ingredients:

4 tbsp. olive oil

2 tbsp. garlic, minced

2 cups leeks, chopped

2 cups carrots, chopped into rounds

2 cups potatoes, diced

2 cups green beans, broken into pieces

Pinch of salt

8 cups vegetable stock

4 cups tomatoes, chopped

½ tsp ground black pepper

2 tsp lemon juice, freshly squeezed

¼ cup parsley, chopped

Directions:

Pour olive oil in a heavy pot. Saute garlic for 2 minutes or until fragrant. Add in leeks, carrots, potatoes, green beans, and salt. Cook for 10 minutes or until just tender. Stir occasionally.

Pour vegetable stock. Add in tomatoes and black pepper. Reduce the heat and allow to simmer for 25 minutes.

Remove from heat. Adjust seasoning, if needed.

To serve, garnish with lemon juice and parsley. serve
    warm.

Vegetable Stock

Ingredients:

1 tbsp. olive oil

8 garlic cloves, minced

1 onion, chopped

2 carrots, chop into chunks

2 celery stalks with leaves

6 thyme sprigs

8 parsley sprigs

2 bay leaves

8 cups water

1 tsp. salt

Directions:

Pour olive oil in a pot. Add in garlic, onion, carrots, celery, thyme, parsley, and bay leaves. Cook for 10 minutes set over medium heat. Stir mixture frequently.

Pour water. Season with salt. Allow to simmer for 30 minutes. Discard vegetables.

Strain the stock using a fine mesh. Press as much liquid as possible. Discard solids. Adjust seasoning, if needed.

Store in an airtight container. Use as needed. Freeze
leftovers.

Country Cabbage Soup

Ingredients:
1 Tbsp. olive oil

1 white onion, sliced

1 russet potato, diced

½ celery stalk, chopped

1 carrot, sliced

1 tomato, diced

2 ½ cups vegetable stock

2 cups green cabbage leaves, shredded

Pinch of sea salt

Pinch of ground black pepper, to taste

Directions:
Pour olive oil in a soup pot. Once hot, sauté white onion for 2 minutes or until tender. Add in carrot, tomato, potato, cabbage, and celery. Pour vegetable broth. Stir well to combine.

Bring mixture to a boil. Once boiling, reduce to a simmer for 30 minutes or until potatoes are tender. Season with salt and pepper.

To serve, ladle soup bowls. Serve warm.

Salad

Two Bean and Avocado Salad

Ingredients:
1 red onion, diced

7 ½ oz canned kidney beans, rinsed, drained

7 ½ oz canned black beans, rinsed, drained

1 red bell pepper, chopped

1 tomato, diced

1tbsp. olive oil

2 Tbsp. lime juice, freshly squeezed

¼ tsp. garlic powder

Pinch of salt

Cayenne pepper, to taste

¼ tsp. chili powder

2 Tbsp. cilantro, chopped

1 avocado, diced

Directions:
Combine onion, kidney beans, black beans, red bell pepper, and tomato in a mixing bowl.

Put together olive oil, lime juice, garlic powder, salt, cayenne pepper, and chili powder in another bowl. Mix well.

Pour dressing over the bean mixture. Toss to coat. Fold in cilantro. Stir.

Place inside the fridge, covered for 1 hour before serving.

To serve, garnish with diced avocado.

Butternut Pumpkin and Spinach Salad

Ingredients:

1 butternut pumpkin, cut to several slices.

1 ½ cups baby spinach leaves

1/4 cup olive oil

1 tbsp. wholegrain mustard

2 tbsp. red wine vinegar

1/2cup feta cheese

3 red onions

Directions:

Preheat the barbecue grill to medium.

Brush butternut pumpkin with olive oil. Season with salt and pepper.

Grill pumpkin slices until tender. Transfer to a plate.

Grill onions until they become translucent. Transfer to a bowl.

Add grilled pumpkin and onion, spinach leaves, and feta cheese in a serving bowl.

For the dressing, combine olive oil, mustard, and vinegar. Stir well. Pour contents into a jar with a tight-fitting lid.

To serve, garnish salad with feta cheese. Drizzle in just the right amount of dressing.

Kidney and Garbanzo Beans Salad

Ingredients:
For the Dressing
    2 Tbsp. apple cider vinegar

    2 Tbsp. extra virgin olive oil

    1 Tbsp. lemon juice, freshly squeezed

    ¼ tsp. paprika

----

    1 red onion, chopped

    7.5 oz. canned kidney beans, rinsed, drained

    ¼ cup black olives, sliced

    7.5 oz. canned garbanzo beans, rinsed, drained

    ½ Tbsp. flat leaf parsley, chopped

    Pinch of salt, to taste

    Pinch of ground black pepper, to taste

Directions:
    For the dressing, mix apple cider vinegar, olive oil, lemon
        juice, and paprika. Whisk well.

    Mix red onion, kidney beans, black olives, garbanzo beans,
        and parsley in a mixing bowl. Drizzle in dressing. Toss
        well to coat.

Season with salt and pepper to taste. Place inside the
fridge, covered for 1 hour before serving. Best served
chilled.

Mixed Greens and Blueberries Salad

Ingredients:

1/4 cup Walnuts, toasted

2 cups fresh blueberries

4 cups mixed salad greens

Vinaigrette dressing- *can be store bought just make sure the ingredients are RA-compliant*

1/2 cup Gorgonzola cheese – *this French blue cheese is allowed in the RA diet*

Directions:

Combine mixed greens, blueberries, walnuts, and cheese in a bowl.

Drizzle in just the right amount of dressing all over salad. Toss well.

Transfer to a plate. Place crumbled Gorgonzola cheese and fresh blueberries on top. Serve.

Spinach and Strawberries Salad

Ingredients:

- 2 bags baby spinach
- 1 small bag strawberries
- 1/4 red onion
- 1 package blue cheese
- 1/2 cup toasted almonds
- Apple cider vinegar, for drizzling
- Pinch of salt
- Pinch of pepper

Directions:

Mix baby spinach, strawberries, red onions, blue cheese, and almonds in a salad bowl.

Drizzle in apple cider vinegar. Season with salt and pepper. Toss well to coat.

Garnish with crumbled blue cheese. Serve.

Kale and Seeds Salad

Ingredients:
For the Dressing

> 1 Tbsp. grape seed oil
>
> 1 ½ Tbsp. apple cider vinegar
>
> ¾ Tbsp. pure maple syrup
>
> 1 garlic clove, crushed
>
> 2 Tbsp. pomegranate juice
>
> Pinch of sea salt
>
> Pinch of ground black pepper, to taste

> 1 apple, cubed
>
> 1 green onion, chopped
>
> 3 cups baby kale, chopped
>
> 3 Tbsp. pomegranate seeds
>
> 3 Tbsp. sunflower seeds
>
> 3 Tbsp. blanched almonds, toasted, slivered

Directions:
Combine grape seed oil, apple cider vinegar, pure maple syrup, garlic clove, pomegranate juice, salt, and ground black pepper in a bottle with tight-fitting lid. Shake vigorously to combine ingredients. Set aside.

Place kale, sunflower seeds, almonds, pomegranate seeds, and green onion in a salad bowl. Toss to combine.

Drizzle in dressing over salad. Toss well to coat. Season with salt and pepper. Serve.

Plant-based Dishes

Spiced Eggplant
Ingredients:
2 eggplant, quartered

Pinch of sea salt

1/3 cup vegetable broth

1 Tbsp. organic soy sauce

2 tsp. rice vinegar

½ tsp. brown sugar

1 ½ Tbsp. apple cider vinegar

2 Tbsp. olive oil

1 garlic clove, chopped

½ tsp. ginger, grated

½ Tbsp. chili bean paste

Directions:
Place eggplant in a colander. Sprinkle with salt. Toss well. Set aside for 30 minutes. Drain on paper towels.

Meanwhile, pour vegetable broth in a bowl. Add in soy sauce, rice vinegar, brown sugar, and apple cider vinegar. Whisk. Set aside.

Pour olive oil in a wok. Once hot, cook eggplant slices. Stir fry until tender. Drain on paper towels. Set aside.

Sauté garlic, ginger, chili bean paste, and the vegetable stock mix. Put back eggplant into the work. Cook for 3 minutes or until the sauce thickens.

Transfer to a serving dish. Serve.

Vegan Chili

Ingredients:

3 Tbsp. olive oil

1 1/4 cups onion, chopped

2 bell peppers, diced

3 garlic cloves, minced

42 oz jarred diced tomatoes, reserve juice

25 oz canned kidney beans, drained, rinsed

1 1/2 tsp sea salt

3 bay leaves

1/6 tsp cayenne pepper

1 1/2 tsp ground cumin

3 tsp chili powder

1 avocado, sliced into cubes

Directions:

Pour olive oil in a stock pot. Saute onion, garlic, and bell peppers for 3 minutes or until translucent and fragrant.

Add in tomatoes and juice, kidney beans, cayenne pepper, ground cumin, chili powder, salt, and bay leaves. Bring to a boil. Once boiling, reduce to a simmer for 40 minutes.

Discard the bay leaves.

To serve, ladle into bowls. Garnish with avocado cubes.

Spiced Oriental Greens

Ingredients:
For the Dressing
- 1/2 tsp garlic cloves, minced
- 1/2 Tbsp. ginger, grated
- 1 scallion, chopped
- 1 Tbsp. olive oil
- 1 Tbsp. toasted sesame oil
- 1 tsp pure maple syrup
- 2 Tbsp. tamari
- 1 Tbsp. black sesame seeds
- 1 Tbsp. white sesame seeds
- 1/3 tsp crushed red chili flakes
- 1 1/4 Tbsp. fresh cilantro, chopped
- 3/4 Tbsp. lime juice, freshly squeezed

- 4 cups Napa cabbage, chopped
- 4 cups red chard, chopped
- 4 cups green chard, chopped

Directions:
1. For the dressing, put together garlic, ginger, scallions, olive oil, sesame oil, maple syrup, tamari, black and white sesame seeds, red chili flakes, cilantro, and lime juice in a bowl.

2. Meanwhile, in a saucepan, pour water. Bring to a boil. Add in red and green chard and Napa cabbage. Cook for 30 seconds or until wilted. Drain.

3. Transfer to a bowl. Pour sauce all over. Toss to coat. Serve.

Sautéed Baby Zucchini

Ingredients:

Pinch of salt

Pinch of pepper

Oregano

1 pack baby zucchini, chopped in half

1 garlic clove, crushed

1 tbsp. olive oil

Directions:

Season baby zucchini with salt and pepper.

Meanwhile, pour olive oil in a non-stick skillet. Slide zucchini. Add in oregano. Cook for 2 minutes on each side. Add the garlic and cook for another minute before serving.

Baked Pineapple with Rice and Veggies
Ingredients:

1 1/2 Tbsp. olive oil

1 1/2 Tbsp. sesame oil, toasted

1/3 cup red onion, minced

1 large pineapple, halved, flesh chopped

3 Tbsp. tamari

3 Tbsp. sweet chili sauce

12 oz extra firm tofu, drain, sliced into cubes

4 1/2 cups brown rice, cooked

3/4 cup carrots, cooked

Pinch of sea salt

Pinch of ground black pepper

Olive oil, for greasing

Directions:

Preheat the oven to 325 degrees F. Cut out sheets of aluminium foil to wrap pineapple shells. Make sure to leave a small opening in the center.

Lightly grease the inner sides with olive oil. Set aside.

Pour olive oil in a wok. Cook tofu cubes until golden brown. Stir in red onion and sauté until translucent.

Add in sesame oil, tamari, and chili sauce. Allow to simmer. Tip in carrots, rice, and corn. Season with salt and pepper. Saute for another 3 minutes.

Add pineapples. Turn off the heat.

Place rice mixture into pineapple shells. Wrap in aluminium foil. Place shells on a baking sheet. Bake for 30 minutes.

Remove from the oven. Unwrap pineapples. Serve immediately.

Vegetable Relish

Ingredients:

2/3 cup red onion, chopped

1 garlic clove, finely chopped

1 avocado, pitted

15 oz can black beans, rinsed

¼ cup fresh cilantro, chopped

3 tbsp. lime juice

1 tbsp. olive oil

Directions:

Place red onion, garlic, avocado, black beans, cilantro, lime juice, and olive oil in a bowl. Mix until all ingredients are combined.

Cover and place inside the fridge to chill for 1 hour or until ready to serve.

Quinoa-Stuffed Bell Peppers

Ingredients:
  3 red bell peppers, halved

  3 green bell peppers, halved

  Pinch of sea salt

  2/3 tsp cayenne pepper

  Olive oil

  1 1/2 cups quinoa, rinsed

  3 cups vegetable stock

For the Stuffing
  4 1/4 Tbsp. olive oil

  3 garlic cloves, minced

  1 onion, minced

  3 celery stalks, minced

  1 carrot, minced

  3/4 tsp cumin

  1 1/2 tsp chili powder

  1/4 cup pumpkin seeds, shelled

  4 Tbsp. basil, chopped

  4 Tbsp. oregano, chopped

  Pinch of salt

  3/4 cup vegetable stock

Directions:

Preheat the oven to 400 degrees F. Place red and green bell peppers on a baking sheet. Season with salt and cayenne pepper. Drizzle in olive oil.

Place quinoa in a saucepan. Pour vegetable stock. Bring to a boil.

Once boiling, reduce to a simmer for 30 minutes, or until the liquid is completely absorbed. Set aside.

Place bell peppers in the oven and bake for 15 minutes.

Meanwhile, heat the olive oil in a skillet. Sauté garlic, onion, celery, carrot, cumin, chili powder, and pumpkin seeds until golden brown.

Add in quinoa into the skillet. Fold in basil. Season with salt. Sauté until combined.

Coat a casserole dish with olive oil. Set aside.

Stuff peppers with filling. Place on the casserole dish. Pour vegetable stock all over stuffed bell peppers. Cover with aluminum foil.

Place inside the oven and bake for 25 minutes. Serve warm.

Mung Beans and Tomato Lettuce Wraps

Ingredients:

2 tbsp. olive oil

2 garlic cloves, diced

1 tomato, diced

1 red bell pepper, sliced

¼ cup mung bean sprouts

1 ½ Tbsp. pumpkin seeds, crushed

½ Tbsp. apple cider vinegar

3 lettuce leaves

1 ½ Tbsp. lemon juice, freshly squeezed

Directions:

Heat olive oil in a non-stick skillet. Once hot, sauté garlic, tomato, bell pepper, mung bean sprouts, and pumpkin seeds. Squeeze in lemon juice. Stir well.

Pour apple cider vinegar into the sprouts. Cook until the garlic is fragrant. Turn off the heat.

Spread lettuce leaves out. Place an equal amount of the veggie mix among them. Roll up lettuce leaves. Serve.

Baked Zucchini with Mint

Ingredients:

2 tbsp. fresh mint leaves

¼ cup lemon juice

1 red onion, sliced thinly

1 tbsp. olive oil

1 tbsp. lemon rind, grated

4 zucchini, halved lengthwise, chopped

Directions:

Preheat the oven at 220 degrees F.

Put together olive oil, onion, zucchini, lemon rind, and lemon juice. Season with salt and pepper.

Toss to combine. Place inside the oven and roast for 20 minutes until tender. Placc mint leaves on top. Serve.

Toasted Sesame Kale

Ingredients:
1 1/2 tsp sesame oil, toasted

3 tsp. olive oil

1 1/2 tsp. garlic, minced

1 1/2 Tbsp. ginger, minced

2 bunches kale, stems chopped off, minced

1 1/2 Tbsp. tamari

1 1/2 Tbsp. sesame seeds

Directions:
Heat sesame and olive oils in a wok set over medium flame. Sauté garlic and ginger for 2 minutes.

Stir in chopped kale stems. Sauté until tender. Add in chopped kale leaves. Sauté until the leaves are wilted. Pour tablespoons of water to prevent kale from burning.

Add in tamari and sesame seeds. Stir well. Serve right away.

Chilli Sweet Potatoes

Ingredients:

3 sweet potatoes, cubed

2 tbsp. olive oil

¼ tsp cayenne pepper

2 tbsp. brown sugar

1 tsp chilli powder

½ tsp salt

Directions:

Preheat the oven to 400 degrees F.

Place sweet potatoes and olive oil in a sealable bag.

Season with cayenne pepper, brown sugar, chilli powder, and salt. Toss well to coat well.

Transfer mix to the baking dish. Place inside the oven and bake for 45 minutes, uncovered. Stir mixture every 15 minutes. Serve.

Pickle and Potato Wraps with Miso Tahina Sauce

Ingredients:
1 onion, diced

3 garlic cloves, chopped

¾ tsp. garlic powder

1 potato, sliced into cubes

3 cups cauliflower florets, chopped

1 ½ Tbsp. tamari

¼ tsp. ground coriander

¾ tsp. cumin

1/3 cup vegetable broth

Pinch of sea salt

1/3 tsp. ground black pepper

Cayenne pepper, to taste

Sweet paprika, to taste

For the Sauce

1 garlic clove

¾ tsp. dried onion flakes

¾ Tbsp. white miso paste

1/3 tsp. cumin powder

Cayenne pepper, to taste

1/3 cup tahini

3 Tbsp. water

1 ½ Tbsp. apple cider vinegar

¾ Tbsp. lemon juice, freshly squeezed

Freshly ground black pepper, to taste

----

3 whole wheat tortillas

1 ½ cups romaine lettuce, chopped

3 dill pickle spears

1 ½ Tbsp. flat leaf parsley, chopped

Directions:
Preheat the oven to 425 degrees F.

Combine onion, garlic, garlic powder, potato, cauliflower, tamari, coriander, cumin, and vegetable broth. Season with salt, black pepper, cayenne, and sweet paprika in a mixing bowl. Mix well.

Spread mixture in a baking dish. Place inside the oven and
  bake for 40 minutes, stirring once after 20 minutes.

To make the sauce, garlic, dried onion flakes, white miso
  paste, cumin powder, cayenne pepper, tahini, water,
  apple cider vinegar, lemon juice, and black pepper in a
  food processor. Blend until smooth. Set aside.

Take baking dish out of the oven. Set aside.

Warm whole wheat tortillas. Spread sauce. Divide
  vegetable filling among tortillas. Add dill pickle spear
  and scatter parsley on top. Roll up. Serve right away.

Arugula, Endive, and Radicchio Salad with Garlic Dressing

Ingredients:

- 1 bunch arugula

- 1 head endive

- 1 head radicchio

- 4 tsp. vegetable oil

- 1 garlic clove, minced

- 1/2 cup of plain yogurt, fat-free

- 1 tbsp. apple cider vinegar

- 1 tbsp. organic honey

- 1/2 tsp. salt

- Pinch of ground pepper

Directions:
1. In a platter, place arugula, endive, and radicchio.

2. To make the dressing, combine vegetable oil, garlic, yogurt, apple cider vinegar, honey, salt, and pepper in the blender. Process until smooth.

3. Drizzle dressing all over salad. Garnish with chives before serving.

Barley Vegetable Soup

Ingredients:
1 Tbsp. olive oil

1 onion, chopped

1 carrot, sliced

1 celery rib, chopped

½ cup barley, uncooked

7 oz. diced tomatoes

¼ cup garbanzo beans

¼ tsp. dried parsley

¼ tsp. dried thyme

Pinch of sea salt

Pinch of ground black pepper

4 cups vegetable stock

1 bay leaf

Directions:

1. Pour olive oil in a soup pot set over medium heat. Sauté onion, carrots, and celery for 3 minutes or until tender.

2. Add in barley, diced tomatoes, garbanzo beans, dried parsley, dried thyme, salt, black pepper, vegetable stock, and bay leaf.

3. Bring mixture to a simmer, covered for 20 minutes. Discard bay leaf.

4. To serve, ladle soup in bowls.

Sweet Potato Casserole

Ingredients:

4 cups sweet potato, cubed

2 eggs, beaten

4 tbsp. butter, softened

1 cup packed brown sugar, divided

½ tsp salt

½ tsp vanilla extract

½ cup milk

1/3 cup Buckwheat flour

½ cup pecans, chopped

Directions:

Preheat the oven to 325 degrees.

Place sweet potatoes in a saucepan. Pour water. Cook until the potatoes are fork tender. Drain and then mash.

Put together eggs, butter, mashed sweet potato, half of the sugar, salt, vanilla and milk. Whisk until smooth. Transfer to a baking dish.

Combine Buckwheat flour and brown sugar in a bowl. Add in butter. Stir mixture until coarse. Fold in pecans.

Spread on top of the sweet potato. Place inside the oven and bake for 30 minutes.

Roasted Squash with Cranberries

Ingredients:
1 butternut squash, peeled, halved, seeds removed, sliced into cubes

1 1/2 Tbsp. olive oil

1/4 tsp ground nutmeg

1 tsp. sea salt

1/4 tsp ground black pepper

1/4 tsp dried sage

1 onion, sliced into wedges

1/4 cup dried cranberries

Non-stick cooking spray

Directions:
Preheat the oven to 400 degrees F. Lightly grease a baking sheet with nonstick cooking spray.

Drizzle in olive oil over squash. Sprinkle with nutmeg, salt, black pepper, and sage. Add in onions. Toss well.

Spread squash on a baking sheet. Roast for 30 minutes, stirring often to prevent burning.

Remove baking sheet from the oven. Add in cranberries. Serve right away.

Spiced Stir Fry Eggplant

Ingredients:
1 eggplant, sliced

Pinch of sea salt

2 tsp. rice vinegar

1/3 cup vegetable broth

1 Tbsp. organic soy sauce

1 ½ Tbsp. Chinese cooking wine

2 Tbsp. olive oil

1 garlic clove, chopped

½ tsp. ginger, grated

½ Tbsp. chili bean paste

½ tsp. light brown sugar

Directions:
Place eggplant slices in a colander. Sprinkle salt all over.
  Toss. Let sit for 30 minutes.
Blot eggplants with paper towels. Set aside.
Meanwhile, put together rice vinegar, vegetable broth, soy
  sauce, sugar, and Chinese cooking wine in a bowl.
  Whisk. Set aside.
Pour olive oil in a wok. Sauté eggplant slices until tender.
  Drain on paper towels. Set aside.
In the same wok, sauté garlic, ginger, chili bean paste,
  sugar, and broth mixture.

Put back eggplant into the work. Cook for 2 minutes until
    the sauce is thickens.
Transfer to a serving dish. Serve.

Potato and Cauliflower Kadahi

Ingredients:
1 potato, sliced into chunks

1 Tbsp. coconut oil

2 green chili peppers, sliced

2 garlic cloves, crushed

1 onion, thinly sliced

½ cup cauliflower florets, chopped

½ cup vegetable broth

¼ cup cilantro, chopped

1 ½ Tbsp. lemon juice, freshly squeezed

½ tsp. black mustard seeds, crushed

½ tsp. cumin seeds

4 curry leaves

Pinch of sea salt, to taste

Directions:
Place potato chunks in a saucepan. Bring to a boil until fork tender. Drain. Set aside.

Pour coconut oil in a wok. Sauté green chili peppers until fragrant. Remove and discard.

Add onion into the chili oil followed by curry leaves, cauliflower, mustard seeds, and cumin seeds. Sauté until fragrant.

Stir in garlic, ginger, potatoes, vegetable broth, chili
   powder, and lemon juice. Allow to simmer until the
   liquids are reduced.
Season with salt and cilantro. Stir fry until heated through.
Transfer vegetables to a serving dish. Sprinkle remaining
   cilantro on top.

Tofu Frittata

Ingredients:

1/2 lb extra firm tofu, drained, crumbled

1/2 tsp onion powder

1/2 tsp garlic powder

1/8 tsp turmeric

2 Tbsp. nutritional yeast

3/4 tsp Dijon mustard

Pinch of sea salt

Pinch of ground black pepper

1/2 cup fresh mixed vegetables of choice, chopped

Non-stick cooking spray

Directions:

Preheat the oven to 400 degrees F. Lightly grease a baking pan. Set aside.

Place crumbled tofu in a bowl. Mix in onion and garlic powders, turmeric, nutritional yeast, and Dijon mustard. Season with salt and ground pepper. Mix.

Fold in the chopped vegetables, then pack the mixture into the prepared baking pan.

Bake for 20 minutes or until firm.

Remove from the oven. Transfer to the cooling rack for 3 minutes. Flip over on a platter. Serve.

Fish Recipes
Egg Noodle Tuna Casserole

Ingredients:

7 oz can tuna, juices reserved

4 oz mushrooms, drained

½ cup celery, finely chopped

¾ cup evaporated milk

10 ¼ oz can cream of celery soup

1 tsp. black pepper

½ onion, chopped finely

1 cup cheddar cheese, grated, divided

½ cup mayonnaise

8 oz egg noodles

Directions:

Cook the noodles in salted water until it is al dente. Drain it and keep warm.

Set the oven at 325 degrees. Combine the ingredients in a large dish. Make sure to reserve ½ cup of cheese for topping.

Spread the cheese generously on top.

Bake it for 30 minutes then serve hot.

Mediterranean-Style Tuna Salad

Ingredients:

- 15 oz. albacore tuna in oil, drained, crumbled
- ¾ cup red peppers, roasted, diced
- 1/3 cup green olives, quartered
- 1 ½ Tbsp. capers, drained
- 1 ½ cups feta cheese, crumbled
- ¾ cup extra virgin olive oil
- 1/3 cup fresh parsley, chopped
- 1 ½ Tbsp. lemon juice, freshly squeezed
- Pinch of fine salt
- Pinch of ground black pepper, to taste
- Dash of red pepper flakes
- 1 ½ cups endives, leaves separated

Directions:

1. Place crumbled tuna, roasted red peppers, green olives, capers, feta cheese, olive oil, parsley, and lemon juice in a bowl. Mix well.
2. Season with salt, pepper, and red pepper flakes. Stir.
3. To serve, divide equal amounts of salad in airtight containers. Add in endive leaves. Place inside the fridge, sealed for 30 minutes before serving. This can keep fresh in the fridge for 3 days.

Avocado and Salmon Stuffed Pita Bread
Ingredients:

- 1 wholegrain wheat pita bread, halved

For the tuna
- 1 salmon fillet
- Pinch of sea salt
- Pinch of white pepper, to taste
- Dash of Spanish paprika
- olive oil

For the Fillings
- ¼ shallot, minced
- 1 ripe tomato, minced
- 2 sprigs fresh cilantro leaves, minced
- 1 ripe avocado, minced
- 1 handful iceberg leaves, minced
- 2 Tbsp. lemon juice, freshly squeezed
- Pinch of sea salt
- Pinch of white pepper, to taste

Directions:
1. For the salmon, pour olive oil into non-stick skillet. Season fillet with salt, pepper, and sweet paprika,
2. Fry tuna until golden brown on all sides. Flip often to make for even cooking. Turn off the heat. Let salmon rest for 5 minutes and then flake using a fork.
3. For the filling, put together shallot, tomato, cilantro leaves, avocado, iceberg leaves, lemon juice, salt, and white pepper in a bowl. Toss to combine.

4.   To serve, stuff just the right amount of flaked salmon and fillings into pita breads. Serve.

Spicy Sardine-Stuffed Avocadoes

Ingredients:

1 can sardines in oil, drained
1 tsp. dried pepper flakes
1 tsp. chives, minced, reserve half for garnish
2 Tbsp. mayonnaise, commercial blend is fine as long as it
    is gluten-free, but homemade is better
Dash of turmeric powder
Dash of sweet paprika powder
Pinch of sea salt
Pinch of white pepper
2 ripe avocadoes, halved lengthwise

Directions:

Combine sardines in oil, dried pepper flakes, chives,
    mayonnaise, turmeric powder, sweet paprika powder,
    salt, and white pepper in a mixing bowl. Whisk well.
Adjust taste if needed. Divide into equal portions.
Spoon 1 portion into each avocado cavity. Garnish with
    chives on top. Serve.

Almond Baked Halibut Fillet
Ingredients:

For the halibut
- 2 halibut fillets
- 1 egg, whisked
- ¼ cup wholegrain wheat flour, finely milled
- ¼ cup almond slivers, raw
- Pinch of salt
- Pinch of black pepper, to taste
- olive oil, for greasing

- ⅛ cup cilantro, minced, for garnish

Directions:
1. Preheat the oven to 400°F. Line a baking sheet with parchment paper. Lightly grease with olive oil.
2. Meanwhile, season halibut fillets with salt and pepper. Roll in wheat flour. Dredge into eggs. Coat with almond slivers.
3. Layer fillets on the baking sheet. Place inside the oven and bake for 15 minutes or until the almonds turn golden brown. Remove from the oven. Let sit for 5 minutes.
4. Cool slightly before transferring into the blender. Process until smooth. Season with salt. Process once more.
5. To serve, place 1 halibut fillet on top. Garnish with cilantro.

Tuna and Cucumber Salad

Ingredients:

For the dressing
    1 tsp. English mustard
    1 Tbsp. extra virgin olive oil
    1 Tbsp. apple cider vinegar

For the salad
    1 tsp. extra virgin olive oil
    2 tuna fillets, diced
    4 cups salad greens of choice, divided into equal portions
    2 eggs, quartered
    2 cucumbers, diced into bite-sized pieces
    Pinch of sea salt
    Pinch of black pepper powder

Directions:
    To make the dressing, put together English mustard, olive oil, and apple cider vinegar in a bottle with tight-fitting lid. Shake well to combine. Set aside.
    To make the salad, pour olive oil in a non-stick skillet. Season tuna with salt and pepper. Sear tuna cubes until just golden.
    Transfer to a serving plate. Tent cubes with aluminium foil on top.
    Pour the dressing all over salad greens. Toss to combine.
    Divide into equal portions. Dot equal quantities of eggs, cucumbers, and tuna cubes on top. Serve.

Tuna Salad with Pickle Relish and Cheese

Ingredients:

7 oz can white tuna, flaked

6 tbsp. mayonnaise, preferably homemade, if store-bought, make sure it's gluten-free

1 tbsp. Parmesan cheese

1/8 tsp minced onion flakes, dried

1 pinch garlic powder

¼ tsp curry powder

3 tbsp. sweet pickle relish

1 tsp dried dill weed

1 tbsp. dried parsley

Directions:

Put together tuna and mayonnaise in a bowl. Add in onion flakes and Parmesan cheese.

Season mixture with garlic powder, curry powder, sweet pickle, dill, and parsley. Mix well to combine.

Serve as is or with a gluten-free bread.

Tuna and Avocado Ceviche on Jicama Slices

Ingredients

For ceviche
- 1 shallot, minced
- Pinch of sea salt
- 1 Tbsp. apple cider vinegar
- 1 Tbsp. capers in oil, drained
- ½ cup lemon juice, freshly squeezed
- 1 garlic clove, minced
- 1 green chili, minced
- Pinch of black pepper, to taste
- ¼ cup extra virgin olive oil
- 2 jicama, sliced into thick sized medallions, the rest minced for ceviche
- 1 lb. fresh tuna fillet, diced into bite-sized pieces
- 1ripe avocado, diced into bite-sized pieces

Directions:

Add in shallot and salt in a bowl. Set aside for 30 minutes. Rinse under running water. Squeeze out excess moisture. Drain.

Place shallot in a mixing bowl. Pour apple cider vinegar, capers, lemon juice, garlic, green chili, black pepper, and olive oil. Mix gently.

Add in jicama, tuna, and avocadoes when ready to serve. Toss to combine.

Divide into equal portions.

To serve, spoon just the right amount of ceviche on chilled jicama slice. Serve.

Sardine and Garden Salad

Ingredients:
- 2 tomatoes, diced
- 2 cups arugula leaves, chopped
- 1 cucumber, diced
- 1 red onion, minced
- 2 sardine fillets in oil, chopped
- 2 sardine fillets in oil, drained
- ¼ cup fresh flat leaf parsley, chopped

For the dressing
- ½ Tbsp. lemon juice, freshly squeezed
- Pinch of sea salt
- Pinch of ground black pepper, to taste
- 2 Tbsp. extra virgin olive oil

Directions:
1. Put together lemon juice, salt, ground black pepper, and olive oil in a bowl. Mix well. Set aside.
2. Toss tomatoes, arugula leaves, onion, tomatoes, and parsley in a salad bowl. Add in sardines. Mix well.
3. To serve, divide sardine fillets into individual servings. Drizzle in dressing over salad. Serve. This can keep for 3 days in the fridge.

Citrus Tuna Steaks

Ingredients:

4 4oz tuna steaks

1 garlic clove, minced

½ tsp oregano, chopped

¼ cup light soy sauce

1 tbsp. lemon juice

¼ cup orange juice

½ tsp ground black pepper

2 tbsp. parsley, chopped

2 tsp. olive oil

Directions:

Preheat the grill to high heat.

Put together garlic, oregano, light soy sauce, lemon juice, orange juice, pepper, parsley, and olive oil in a bowl.

Add in tuna steaks into the marinade mixture. Place inside the fridge for 30 minutes to 1 hour to marinate.

Spread oil on the grill. Grill tuna steak for 5 minutes. Turn and baste with the remaining marinade.

Cook for 5 minutes until cooked to your desired doneness. Serve.

Mackerel on Cucumber Sandwich

Ingredients:
For the filling
    1 tsp. olive oil
    1 6 oz. mackerel fillet, sliced into thin matchsticks
    4 Kalamata olives, minced
    4 cherry tomatoes, deseeded
    1 tsp. capers in brine
    1 jalapeño pepper, minced
    Pinch of white pepper
    Pinch of sea salt

For the sandwich
    2 cucumbers, halved lengthwise, seeds scooped out, chill
        before using
    2 Tbsp. apple cider vinegar, divided
    1 head red leaf lettuce, shredded, chill before using
    1 lime, quartered

Directions:
To make the filling, pour olive oil into the saucepan. Cook mackerel fillets until browned. Transfer to plate. Tent with aluminium foil.

In the same pan, cook Kalamata olives, cherry tomatoes, and capers until tomatoes are a little tender and wilted. Turn off the heat

Add in jalapeño pepper, salt6t, and pepper. Stir well.

To serve, drizzle in ½ tablespoon of apple cider vinegar on each cucumber half. Place equal amounts of lettuce.

Add mackerel tomato-capers mix on lettuce leaves. Serve with lime quarters.

Tuna and Tomatoes Bread

Ingredients:

1 tbsp. Dijon mustard

1 tbsp. olive oil

2 tsp fresh lemon juice

2 tbsp. green onions, thinly sliced, divided

1/8 tsp salt

¼ tsp black pepper

5 oz can white tuna in water, drained, flaked

2 Whole wheat bread, toasted, halved lengthwise, carve hallow at the top and bottom part, leave at least 1 inch thick shell, set aside torn bread

4 ¼ inch plum tomatoes, sliced

2 tsp green onions, thinly sliced

Directions:

Prepare the broiler.

Put together Dijon mustard, olive oil, lemon juice, green onions, salt, and pepper in a bowl. Mix well. Add in tuna.

Place bread cut side up in a baking sheet. Broil until toasted.

Spoon tuna mixture into the bread. Place tomato slices on
top.

Broil for another 2 minutes. Garnish with green onion.
Serve.

Seared Tuna

Ingredients:

¼ cup rice wine vinegar

2 garlic cloves, chopped

2 tsp sambal oelek, gluten free

½ cup light soy sauce

4 scallion greens, for garnish

1 ½ inch ginger, grated

4 scallions, white and green parts chopped finely

Olive oil

4 6 oz tuna steaks

Directions:

Mix rice vinegar, garlic, sambal oelek, light soy sauce, scallions, and ginger. Mix well. Add in tuna. Roll and make sure everything is well-coated.

Place inside the fridge, covered for 2 hours to marinate.

Pat tuna to with paper towel to remove excess liquid at room temperature.

Pour olive oil in a large pan. Once the oil is hot, remove from heat and then cook tuna for 1 minute on each side.

Slice and then transfer to a platter. Sprinkle dark greens on top before serving.

Salmon and Dill Spread

Ingredients:

- 4 oz. smoked salmon
- 4 oz. non- fat cream cheese
- 2 ½ Tbsp. mayonnaise
- Pinch of sea salt
- Pinch of ground black pepper, to taste
- 2 Tbsp. fresh dill, chopped

Directions:

1. Place smoked salmon, mayonnaise, and cream cheese in a food processor. Pulse until all ingredients are well-combined.
2. Pour mixture into an airtight container. Add in fresh dill. Season with salt and pepper.
3. Place inside the fridge for a few hours or until ready to serve. This spread is best served with cucumber, carrot, and celery sticks.

Sesame Seared Tuna with Wasabi

Ingredients:

2 tbsp. sesame oil

1 tbsp. honey

1 tbsp. mirin

¼ cup light soy sauce

1 tbsp. rice wine vinegar

½ cup sesame seeds

4 6 oz tuna steaks

1 tbsp. olive oil

Wasabi paste

Directions:

Combine sesame oil, honey, mirin, and soy sauce in a bowl. Mix well. Pour rice vinegar.

Coat tuna steaks with the soy mixture. Spread sesame seeds on a plate. Roll steaks in the sesame seeds. Press down firmly to coat.

Pour olive oil in a pan. Sear tuna steaks and cook for 30 seconds on each side. Serve with the wasabi.

Food with Fruit Ingredients

Anchovy on Avocado and Salad Greens

Ingredients:

For the dressing

- 1 tsp. English mustard
- Pinch of sea salt
- Pinch of black pepper powder
- 1 Tbsp. extra virgin olive oil
- 1 Tbsp. lemon juice, freshly squeezed

For the salad

4 cups salad greens of choice

1 can anchovy fillets on olive oil, drained, reserve some oil
   for dressing

1 avocado, just ripe, halved, sliced thinly

2eggs, hard-boiled, quartered

Directions:

1. To make the dressing, mix English mustard, salt, black pepper powder, olive oil, and lemon juice in a bottle with tight-fitting lid. Shake well to mix. Set aside.
2. Pour dressing all over salad greens. Toss well to combine.
3. To serve, divide salad into plates. Dot equal amounts of anchovies, avocadoes, and eggs on top. Serve.

Baked Apricot Oatmeal

Ingredients:

1 ¼ cups almond milk, divided

½ cup rolled oats

1/8 tsp. ginger, ground

¼ tsp. ground cinnamon

3 Tbsp. almond butter

¼ cup dried apricots, chopped

¼ tsp. orange zest, grated

Pinch of salt, to taste

2 ½ Tbsp. orange juice, freshly squeezed

Directions:

1. Preheat the oven to 350 degrees F. Prepare a ramekin. Set aside.

2. Pour 1 cup of almond milk into the saucepan. Add in rolled oats. Set aside.

3. Pour almond milk and oats in a sauce pan. Bring to a boil. Once boiling, reduce to a simmer until the oats are tender.

4. Add in ginger, cinnamon, almond butter, dried apricots, orange zest, and salt. Mix well. Turn off the heat.

5. Stir in orange juice and the remaining almond milk. Mix.

6. To serve, pour mixture into the ramekin. Place inside the oven and bake for 10 minutes.

Tuna and Mango Salad

Ingredients:

For the dressing

- ¼ tsp. raw, unprocessed honey
- 3 Tbsp. lemon juice, freshly squeezed
- Pinch of sea salt
- Pinch of black pepper, to taste

- ½ cup, tuna fillet, sliced into cubes, precooked
- 1 ripe mango, diced
- 1 cup red oak leaf lettuce, torn
- ½ cup watercress, torn
- 2 cups round leaf lettuce, torn
- 1 fresh jalapeno pepper, minced

Directions:

1. For the dressing, pour honey, lemon juice, salt, and black pepper in a bowl. Whisk until the salt dissolves.
2. For the salad, combine tuna fillet, diced mango, red oak leaf lettuce, watercress, round leaf lettuce, and jalapeno pepper in a salad bowl. Toss to combine.
3. Drizzle in just the right amount of dressing. Toss to coat.
4. To serve, ladle equal amount of salad on plates. Drizzle in remaining dressing. Serve.

Berry Loaded Salad

Ingredients:

For the dressing

- 3 Tbsp. lemon juice, freshly squeezed
- Pinch of sea salt
- Pinch of black pepper, to taste
- 1 tsp. dried pepper flakes

- 4 endive leaves, chopped to bite-sized pieces
- 2 cups iceberg lettuce, chopped into bite-sized pieces
- 2 fresh strawberries, quartered
- 2 red grapes, seedless, halved
- 2 green grapes, seedless halved
- ¼ cup fresh blueberries, hulled
- 4cherry tomatoes, quartered
- 1 leek, sliced into half-inch pieces
- ½ tsp. raisins
- ½ tsp. almond slivers, toasted

Directions:

1. For the dressing, pour lemon juice, salt, black pepper, and dried pepper flakes in a small bowl. Whisk until the salt dissolves. Adjust taste, if needed.
2. For the salad, combine endive leaves, iceberg lettuce, strawberries, red grapes, green grapes, blueberries, cherry tomatoes, leek, and raisins in a salad bowl. Toss well to combine. Drizzle in half the dressing. Toss to coat.
3. To serve, ladle equal amounts of salad on plates. Drizzle in the remaining dressing. Scatter almond slivers on top. Serve.

Blueberries in Cream Cheese Flapjacks

Ingredients:

- 2 eggs
- 2 cream cheese
- Dash of nutmeg powder
- Dash of pinch cinnamon powder
- ⅛ tsp. honey
- coconut oil, for greasing

For garnish

- ½ cup frozen blueberries or any seasonal berries, thawed

Directions:

1. Whisk eggs, cream cheese, nutmeg powder, cinnamon powder, and honey until well-combined.
2. Pour coconut oil in a non-stick skillet. Place just the right amount of batter mix into the pan. Cook until the edges are set and the center bubbling. Add half of the berries in the center.
3. Flip the other side. Transfer to a plate. Repeat step for the remaining batter.
4. To serve, stack flapjacks on a plate.

Granola Fruits and Nuts

Ingredients:
- 4 cups old-fashioned rolled oats

- 1/2 cup almond slivers

- 1/4 cup sesame seeds

- 1 tsp. cinnamon

- 1/8 tsp. nutmeg

- 1/4 tsp. salt

- 1/3 cup honey

- 2 tbsp. olive oil

- 1 tsp. vanilla extract

- 2 tbsp. warm water

- 6 tbsp. maple syrup

- 1 cup golden raisins

- 1 cup dried cranberries

Directions:
1. Preheat the oven to 300 degrees. Lightly grease a jelly-roll pan with oil.

2. Combine rolled oats, almonds, sesame seeds, cinnamon, nutmeg, and salt in a bowl. Mix well.

3. Put together honey, olive oil, vanilla extract, water, and maple syrup in another bowl. Pour over the oats mixture. Toss well to combine.

4. Spread mixture over a jelly-roll pan. Place inside the oven and bake for 55 minutes. Stir well breaking large clumps every 10 minutes.

5. Take out pan from the oven and add in raisins and cranberries. Store in an airtight container and store leftovers in the fridge.

Red Berries Smoothie
Ingredients:

- ½ cup frozen cranberries
- ½ cup frozen raspberries
- 4strawberries, cubed
- 2 overripe banana, cubed
- ½ cup crushed ice
- ½ tsp. honey raw, unprocessed

Directions:

1. Place cranberries, raspberries, strawberries, banana, crushed ice, and honey in a blender. Process until smooth.
2. To serve, pour in tall glasses. Serve immediately.

Vegetable Power Juice

Ingredients:
- 2 ripe tomatoes, chopped
- 1 pear, chopped
- 1 cucumber, chopped
- 1 lime, sliced into wedges
- ½ cup crushed ice

Directions:
1. Place tomatoes, pear, cucumber, lime, and crushed ice in a blender. Process until smooth.
2. To serve, pour in tall glasses. Serve immediately.

Lime Water Infused with Strawberries and Grapes

Ingredients:

- 1 cup strawberries, hulled, sliced thinly
- 2 cups red grapes, seedless, halved
- 1 lime, sliced into thick half-moons
- 1½ cups water
- 1 cup crushed ice
- ¼ tsp. raw, unprocessed honey

Directions:

1. Place strawberries, red grapes, lime, water, and crushed ice in a tall, lidded pitcher. Seal the lid.
2. Steep for 3 hours. Strain beverage before serving. Add in honey. Serve.

Apple Cinnamon Oatmeal

Ingredients:
 1 cup traditional rolled oats

 2 apples, diced

 1 tsp. ground ginger

 2 tsp. ground cinnamon

 2 Tbsp. chia seeds

 2 cups almond milk, unsweetened

 ¾ cup applesauce

 1 tsp. vanilla bean paste

 2 Tbsp. pure maple syrup

Directions:
 Combine rolled oats, apples, ginger, cinnamon, chia seeds, almond milk, and applesauce in a saucepan. Stir well.

 Cook for 10 minutes whilst stirring frequently. Add in vanilla bean paste. Mix.

 Once cooked, divide oatmeal into bowls. drizzle in maple syrup. Serve.

Berry Cashew French Toast

Ingredients:
3 Tbsp. virgin coconut oil

¾ cup raw cashews

6 strawberries, halved

1/3 cup blueberries

3 Tbsp. pure maple syrup

1/6 tsp. ground cinnamon

1/6 tsp. nutmeg

1 ½ cups almond milk, unsweetened

1 ½ tsp. pure vanilla extract

Pinch of sea salt, to taste

1 ½ cups water

6 wheat bread

3 Tbsp. coconut cream

Directions:
Preheat the grill over medium flame. Lightly grease with coconut oil.

Combine cashews, strawberries, blueberries, maple syrup, water, cinnamon, nutmeg, almond milk, vanilla extract, salt, and water in a blender. Blend until smooth. Transfer to a bowl. Set aside.

Soak each bread slice in the milk mixture. Cook for 1 minute on each side or until golden brown.

Transfer to a platter. Spoon coconut cream on top.

Power Carrot Juice

Ingredients:
- 1 carrot, chopped
- 1 pear, chopped
- 1 red apple, chopped
- 1 sprig fresh mint, for garnish

Directions:
1. Place carrot, pear, and red apple into the juicer. Process until smooth.
2. Pour into tall glass. Garnish with mint on top. Serve.

Tropical Infusion

Ingredients:
- 1 cup pineapples, diced, reserve juice, rinse well
- 2 kiwi fruits, quartered
- 1 ripe mango, cubed
- 1 ripe papaya, cubed
- 4 cups water
- 1 cup ice cubes

Directions:
1. Place pineapples, kiwi, mango, papaya, water, and ice cubes in a large glass pitcher. Stir well.
2. Place inside the fridge to chill for 2 hours or more before serving.
3. Pour into tall glasses to serve.

Peach, Pineapple, and Mango Smoothie
Ingredients:

- 1peach, cubed
- 1 cup pineapple, cubed
- 1 ripe mango, cubed
- 1 cup crushed ice
- ½ tsp. raw, unprocessed honey

Directions:

1. Place peach, pineapple, mango, crushed ice, and honey in a blender. Process until smooth.
2. Divide into glasses. Serve immediately.

Greens with Sunflower Seed Salad

Ingredients:

For the dressing
- 1 tsp. apple cider vinegar
- ½ tsp. Dijon mustard
- ¼ tsp. raw, unprocessed honey
- 2 Tbsp. extra virgin olive oil
- 2 Tbsp. fresh chives, minced
- 1 tsp. lemon juice, freshly squeezed
- Pinch of sea salt
- Pinch of black pepper, to taste

- 4 dandelion greens, torn
- 1 head round lettuce, torn
- ¼ lb. arugula, torn
- 1 red tomato, cubed
- 1 red apple, cubed
- 1 egg, hard-boiled, chopped
- 1 Tbsp. raw, shelled sunflower seeds, roasted

Directions:

1. For the dressing, pour apple cider vinegar, Dijon mustard, honey, olive oil, chives, lemon juice, salt, and black pepper in a small bottle with tight fitting lid. Seal and shake well. Adjust taste, if needed. Set aside.

2. For the salad, place 4 dandelion greens, lettuce, arugula, tomato, apple, and hard-boiled egg into the salad bowl. Toss well to combine. Drizzle in half the dressing. Toss to coat.

3.	To serve, ladle equal amounts of salad on plates. Drizzle in the remaining dressing all over. Scatter sunflower seeds on top. Serve.

Orange Water Infused with Cucumber and Grapes

Ingredients:

- 1 cucumber, halved, sliced into thick half-moons
- 2 cups red grapes, seedless, halved
- 1 sweet orange, halved, sliced into thick half-moons
- 1½ cups water
- 1 cup crushed ice
- ¼ tsp. raw, unprocessed honey

Directions:

1. Place cucumber, red grapes, sweet orange, water, and crushed ice into a tall, lidded pitcher. Seal the lid.
2. Allow to steep for 3 hours or more. Strain before serving.
3. To serve, pour honey into individual glasses.

Piña Colada Smoothie
Ingredients:

- 1 cup crushed pineapple, drained, juices reserved, chilled for 3 hours

- 1/2 cup pineapple juice

- 1 cup coconut water

- 1 cup frozen vanilla yogurt, low-fat

- 1 cup ice cubes

Directions:

1. Thaw chilled pineapple at a room temperature for 10 minutes.

2. Transfer to a blender together pineapple juice, coconut water, frozen yogurt, and ice cubes in a blender.

3. Process until smooth. Serve.

Blueberry and Cashew Salad
Ingredients:

For the dressing
- 2 Tbsp. apple cider vinegar
- 1 Tbsp. blueberries
- ¼ tsp. raw, unprocessed honey
- 2 Tbsp. extra virgin olive oil
- Pinch of sea salt
- Pinch of black pepper, to taste

- 1 head lettuce, torn
- ½ cup baby spinach leaves
- ¼ cup fresh blueberries
- ¼ cup pre-cooked boiled chicken, shredded
- ¼ lb. watercress, torn
- ¼ cup cashew nuts, chopped, toasted

Directions:

1. For the dressing, pour apple cider vinegar, blueberries, honey, extra virgin olive oil, salt, and black pepper into a blender. Process until smooth. Adjust taste, if needed. Set aside.
2. For the salad, place lettuce, baby spinach, blueberries, boiled chicken, watercress, and cashew nuts into the salad bowl.
3. Drizzle in half the dressing. Toss well to combine.
4. To serve, ladle equal amounts of salad on plates. Drizzle in the remaining dressing. Serve.

Snacks and Beverages

Coconut Butter on Vegan Rye Bread

Ingredients:
For the coconut butter
- 1 package coconut flakes, use the high quality

For the Rye Bread
- 2 cups warm water
- 2¼ tsp. active dry yeast

Dry ingredients
- ½ cup dark rye flour, coarsely milled
- 1½ cups dark rye flour, finely milled
- 2 cups bread flour, add more for kneading
- 1 Tbsp. palm sugar, crumbled
- 1¾ tsp. salt
- 3 tsp. black caraway seeds, lightly toasted, reserve some for garnish

Wet ingredients
- 1 Tbsp. pure maple syrup
- olive oil, for greasing

Directions:
1. Preheat the oven to 375°F.
2. To make the coconut butter, put coconut flakes into the blender. Process for 5 minutes or until thick. Transfer to a non-reactive container with lid. Allow mixture to rest butter for 15 minutes.

3. To make the bread, pour water and yeast in a bowl. Whisk well to combine. Set aside for 10 minutes or until frothy.

4. Add in both coarsely and finely milled dark rye flour, bread flour, palm sugar, and salt in a large bowl. mix. Make a well in the center.

5. Pour maple syrup and yeast mixture. Mix the dough until it comes together. Turn out dough on a floured surface. Knead until no longer sticky. Form into a ball.

6. Roll dough in another bowl greases with oil. Cover with saran wrap. Let the dough rise until it doubles in size.

7. Punch dough down. Form into a ball again. Let rise for another 1 ½ hours.

8. Lightly grease a bread loaf pan with oil. Turn out the dough into the loaf pan. Scatter caraway seeds on top. Let it have its final rising for 40 minutes.

9. Place the loaf pan in the middle rack of the oven. Bake for 40 minutes or until golden brown.

10. Remove from the oven. Allow to cool on the cooling rack.

11. Slide out bread from the loaf pan, and then slice. Serve with homemade coconut butter on top.

Baked Eggs in Avocado Halves with Wholegrain Sourdough Bread

Ingredients:

- 2 slices wholegrain sourdough bread

For the eggs

- 1just ripe avocado, halved
- 2 small eggs
- 1 tsp. lemon juice, freshly squeezed
- ½ tsp. fresh chives, minced, for garnish
- ¼ tsp. extra virgin olive oil, for garnish
- Dash of red pepper flakes
- Dash of Spanish paprika powder
- Pinch of sea salt
- Pinch of white pepper, to taste

Directions:

1. Preheat the oven to 350°F.
1. Squeeze in lemon juice on cut sides of avocado halves. Season with paprika powder.
2. Place avocado halves cut-side up on ramekins (or oven-safe bowls) to prevent these from rolling around. Place ramekins on baking sheet.
3. Carefully crack eggs into avocado cavities. Season lightly with red pepper flakes, sea salt and white pepper.
4. Bake avocadoes for 15 minutes or until desired egg yolks doneness is achieved. Remove baking sheet from the oven.

5.   To serve, place cooked avocado and sourdough bread on a plate. Garnish with chives. Drizzle in olive oil.

All Berries Sweetened Oats with Coconut Milk

Ingredients:

For oats

- ½ cup steel cut oats
- 1½ cups water
- Pinch of salt
- ½ cup coconut milk

For the fruits

- ½ cup frozen blueberries
- 1 Tbsp. frozen raspberries
- 1 Tbsp. frozen blackberries
- ½ cup frozen strawberries, quartered

Dircctions:

1. For the oats, place oats, water, and salt into a Dutch oven. Bring mixture to a boil whilst stirring often.

2. Reduce the heat and allow to simmer for 10 minutes with the lid partially on. Turn off the heat.

3. Let oats rest for 3 minutes. Pour coconut milk. Stir.

4.   To make the seasoning, add in blueberries, raspberries, blackberries, and strawberries. Stir mixture and pour over oats.

5.   To serve, ladle into bowls.

Avocado Cream Cheese on Cucumber Slices

Ingredients:

- 1 avocado, flesh scooped out
- 8 oz. cream cheese
- 1 Tbsp. lemon juice, freshly squeezed
- 1 cucumber, sliced into 1/3 inch rounds
- Tabasco sauce, to taste
- 4 oz. red salmon, flaked
- ½ Tbsp. green onion, chopped

Directions:

1. Place avocado flesh in a bowl. Mash avocado. Add in cream cheese. Mix until all ingredients come together. Squeeze in lemon juice. Season with tabasco sauce. Mix.
2. Arrange the cucumber slices on a serving platter. Divide avocado cream cheese mix among cucumber. Add in flaked red salmon.
3. To serve, garnish with green onions on top.

Twice-Baked Sweet Potatoes and Yam Matchsticks

Ingredients:
For the sugar glaze

- ⅛ tsp. cinnamon powder

- 2 Tbsp. brown sugar, crumbled

- ⅛ tsp. nutmeg powder

- 2 Tbsp. olive oil, for drizzling

- 2sweet potatoes, sliced into thick matchsticks

- 1 purple yam, sliced into thick matchstick

- water, for spraying

- Pinch of fine salt

Directions:

1. Preheat the oven to 350°F. Line a baking sheet with parchment paper.

2. To make the glaze, combine cinnamon powder, brown sugar, and nutmeg powder in a bowl. Toss to combine.

3. For the potatoes, place yam and sweet potato matchsticks on the baking sheet. Spray with small amount of water and add a pinch of salt to taste.

4. Place inside the oven and bake for 45 minutes. Remove from the oven.

5.   Drizzle in oil on top of the veggies. Sprinkle sugar glaze. Toss to evenly coat using a pair of tongs.

6.   Return to the oven and cook for another 5 minutes. Turn off the heat.

7.   Place on a cooling rack and allow to cool at room temperature. Serve.

Veggie Fritters

Ingredients:

- 1 cup fresh spinach leaves, julienned
- 1 red onion, julienned
- 1 carrot, grated
- 1 sweet potato, grated
- 1potato, grated
- Pinch of salt
- 1 garlic, grated
- 1½ Tbsp. almond flour
- ¼ tsp. sweet paprika
- 1Tbsp.red pepper flakes
- Pinch of white pepper, to taste
- ½ lime, sliced into 4 wedges, for garnish
- coconut oil, for frying
- ¼ cup chives, minced, for garnish

Directions:

1. Place spinach leaves, onion, carrot, sweet potato, potato, and salt into a cheesecloth. Using your hands, toss veggies to mix.
2. Bundle cheesecloth up and squeeze out as much liquid as possible. Transfer vegetables into a mixing bowl.
3. Add in garlic, almond flour, sweet paprika, red pepper flakes, and white pepper into the bowl. Mix well.
4. Divide into equal fritters. Shape into patties.

5.   Meanwhile, pour coconut oil into a non-stick frying pan over medium heat. Once hot, place 1 fritter and fry until golden brown on one side. Flip. Cook the other side for another 2 minutes.

6.   Drain on paper towels. Repeat until all fritters are cooked. Serve.

Coconut and Mangoes Flapjacks

Ingredients:
- Coconut oil

Dry ingredients
- 1¼ cup whole wheat flour

- ¼ tsp. baking soda

- 1 tsp. baking powder

- ¼ tsp. cinnamon powder

- ¼ tsp. nutmeg powder

- ¼ tsp. all spice powder

- ½ cup desiccated coconut, shredded

- Pinch of salt

Wet ingredients
- ¾ cup coconut water

- ¾ cup coconut milk

- ½ tsp. vanilla extract

For the Toppings
- ½ cup fresh coconut flesh, shredded, divided

- ¼ cup fresh ripe mangoes, divided

Directions:
1. Meanwhile, pour whole wheat flour, baking soda, baking powder, cinnamon powder, nutmeg powder, all

spice powder, desiccated coconut, and salt all into a mixing bowl. Stir. Make a well in the center.

2. Pour coconut water, coconut milk, and vanilla extract into the center. Whisk until all ingredients come together.

3. Add in half of fresh coconut and mangoes. Mix well.

4. Pour coconut oil into a non-stick frying pan. Pour ¼ cup of batter into the pan. Cook until the center is no longer runny and the edges set. Flip. Cook the other side for 1 minute.

5. Transfer to a serving plate. Repeat until the remaining batter is cooked.

6. To serve, stack pancakes. Top with shredded coconut and few pieces of mangoes.

Easy Boiled Plantains

Ingredients:
- 6plantains, preferably overripe

- water, for boiling

Directions:
1. Place plantains in a saucepan set over high heat. Pour just enough water to submerge plantains. Bring to a boil.

2. Reduce the heat with the lid on and cook plantains for15 minutes or until the water changes in color.

3. Turn off the heat. Remove plantains. Discard cooking water.

4. Let cool slightly before serving.

Citrus-Flavored Fruits and Vegetable Kebab

Ingredients:
For the citrus seasoning

- 1 sweet orange, freshly juiced
- ¼ tsp sugar
- Dash of smoked paprika powder
- Pinch of salt
- Pinch of black pepper

For the kebab

- 1 onion, sliced into large wedges
- 8 cherry tomatoes, whole
- 1 apple, cubed
- 1 can button mushrooms, whole, rinsed well, approximately 8 smaller pieces
- 1 zucchini, sliced into ½ inch thick medallions
- ½ green bell pepper, sliced into squares

Directions:

1. Preheat the electric grill for 5 minutes.
2. To prepare, soak bamboo skewers in water for 1 hour before using.
3. For the seasoning, put together sweet orange, sugar, paprika powder, salt, and black pepper in a bowl. Whisk well.
4. Thread equal amounts of onion, cherry tomatoes, apple, button mushrooms, zucchini, and

green bell pepper on bamboo skewers. Season kebabs with prepared seasoning.

5.   Grill for 10 minutes, rotating often or until the tomato skins blister.

6.   Transfer to a plate. Slather more seasoning. Serve.

Spiced Crisp Cauliflower

Ingredients:

- 1/2 cup red onion, minced
- 1/2 tsp garlic, minced
- 1/2 Tbsp. ginger, grated
- 3 cups cauliflower florets, chopped
- 2 Tbsp. olive oil
- 1/4 tsp garam masala
- 1/4 tsp curry powder
- 1/8 tsp red chili flakes, crushed
- 1/4 Tbsp. lemon zest, grated
- 1/4 tsp fennel seeds
- 1 tsp sea salt
- 1/2 tsp ground black pepper
- 2 Tbsp. fresh cilantro, chopped
- Non-stick cooking spray, for greasing

Directions:

1. Preheat the oven to 400 degrees F. Lightly coat a rimmed baking sheet with non-stick cooking spray. Set aside.

2. Meanwhile, mix onion, garlic, ginger, cauliflower, olive oil, garam masala, curry powder, red chili flakes, lemon zest, fennel seeds, salt, and ground black pepper in a bowl. Toss well to combine.

3. Spread cauliflower mixture on the rimmed baking sheet. Place inside the oven and roast for 20 minutes or until the cauliflower is crisp and golden brown.

4. Transfer roasted cauliflower to a serving platter. Garnish with cilantro on top. Serve.

Oats and Dates Energy Bars

Ingredients:
- 3 tsp baking powder
- 2 1/4 cups oats, preferably quick cooking
- 1 1/2 tsp ground cinnamon
- 2 cups whole wheat pastry flour
- Pinch of sea salt
- 1 1/2 cups nut milk, unsweetened
- 1 1/2 cups applesauce, unsweetened
- 3/4 cup organic peanut butter
- 3/4 cup pureed dates
- 1 1/2 tsp pure vanilla extract
- 1/3 cup pure maple syrup

Directions:
1. Preheat the oven to 350 degrees F. Line a baking dish with baking paper. Set aside.
2. Combine baking powder, oats, cinnamon, whole wheat pastry flour, and salt in a large mixing bowl.
3. In another bowl, put together nut milk, applesauce, peanut butter, pureed dates, vanilla extract, and maple syrup. Mix wet ingredients into the dry ingredients.
4. Pour batter into the baking dish, Make sure to pack firmly using a spatula.
5. Place inside the oven and bake for 25 minutes or a toothpick inserted comes out clean.

6. Place on a cooling rack for 25 minutes before slicing
   into bite-sized pieces.

Apples and Chamomile Herbal Infusion

Ingredients:
- 1 green apple, sliced into thick half-moons
- ¼ cup chamomile flowers, tea-grade, approximately 2 mini teabags
- 1 pc. 2-inch long dried cinnamon bark
- 4cups water, freshly boiled

Directions:
1. Pour green apple, chamomile flowers, dried cinnamon bark, and water into a tea press or any heat-safe container.
2. Steep herbal infusion for 8 minutes. Strain. Serve.

Dried Leaves Herbal Infusion

Ingredients:
- ⅛ cup dried hawthorn leaves, tea grade, approx. 1 mini teabag
- ⅛ cup dried blackberry leaves, tea grade, approx. 1 mini teabag
- ⅛ cup dried lemon balm leaves, tea grade, approx. 1 mini teabag
- 4 cups water, freshly boiled
- ⅛ tsp. green stevia

Directions:

1. Pour dried hawthorn leaves, dried blackberry leaves, dried lemon balm leaves, water, and green stevia into tea press or any heat-safe container.

2. Steep herbal infusion for 8 minutes. Strain. Serve.

Strawberry and Flaxseed Shake

Ingredients:

- 2 frozen bananas, overripe

- 1 cup frozen strawberries, halved

- 2 cups coconut milk

- 1 cup ice cubes

- 1 Tbsp. green stevia

- 1½ Tbsp. flaxseed, toasted

Directions:

1. Place bananas, strawberries, coconut milk, ice cubes, and green stevia into the blender. Process until smooth.

2. Pour into tall glasses to. Serve.

Shaved Fruits and Vegetables Infusion

Ingredients:

- 1 zucchini, shaved into flat, thin ribbons using a spiralizer, seeds discarded

- 1 carrot, shaved into flat, thin ribbons using a spiralizer

- 1 green mango, shaved into flat, thin ribbons using a spiralizer

- 1 cucumber, shaved into flat, thin ribbons using a spiralizer

- 1 cup ice cubes

- 4 cups water

Directions:
1. Place zucchini, carrot, green mango, cucumber ribbons, ice cubes, and water into a glass pitcher.

2. Stir lightly using a spoon. Place inside the fridge to chill for 2 hours.

3. Pour into tall glasses. Serve.

Power Berries Juice

Ingredients:
- ¼ cup frozen blueberries

- ¼ cup frozen cranberries

- ¼ cup frozen strawberries

- 1 pear

- 1 sprig fresh mint, for garnish

Directions:
1. Place blueberries, cranberries, strawberries, and pear into the juicer. Process until the mixture is smooth.

2. Pour into a tall glass. Put mint on top. Serve.